This book is intended solely for informational and tracking purposes. It is not a substitute for professional medical advice, diagnosis, or treatment. Always consult a qualified healthcare provider regarding any medical concerns, symptoms, questions, and/or conditions. The publisher, author, and associated contractors assume no responsibility for any decisions made based on the information contained within this book. If you have a medical emergency, seek immediate assistance from a licensed medical professional.

Published by House of Sanchez LLC
HOUSEOFSANCHEZ.COM

DATE: SUN MON TUES WED THUR FRI SAT

BREAKFAST

BLOOD SUGAR (BS): ____ TIME __ : __ AM / PM

Insulin Units: ____ mg/dL Total Carbs: ____ grams

MORNING SNACK

BLOOD SUGAR (BS): ____ TIME __ : __ AM / PM

Insulin Units: ____ mg/dL Total Carbs: ____ grams

LUNCH

BLOOD SUGAR (BS): ____ TIME __ : __ AM / PM

Insulin Units: ____ mg/dL Total Carbs: ____ grams

AFTERNOON SNACK

BLOOD SUGAR (BS): ____ TIME __ : __ AM / PM

Insulin Units: ____ mg/dL Total Carbs: ____ grams

DINNER

BLOOD SUGAR (BS): ____ TIME __ : __ AM / PM

Insulin Units: ____ mg/dL Total Carbs: ____ grams

EVENING SNACK

BLOOD SUGAR (BS): ____ TIME __ : __ AM / PM

Insulin Units: ____ mg/dL Total Carbs: ____ grams

BLOOD SUGAR HIGHS

TIME : AM / PM
BLOOD SUGAR (BS): mg/dL
CORRECTION DOSE: units

KETONES
NEGATIVE TRACE SMALL MODERATE LARGE

TIME : AM / PM
BLOOD SUGAR (BS): mg/dL
CORRECTION DOSE: units

KETONES
NEGATIVE TRACE SMALL MODERATE LARGE

TIME : AM / PM
BLOOD SUGAR (BS): mg/dL
CORRECTION DOSE: units

KETONES
NEGATIVE TRACE SMALL MODERATE LARGE

BLOOD SUGAR LOWS

BLOOD SUGAR (BS): mg/dL TIME : AM / PM
CORRECTED WITH:

BLOOD SUGAR (BS): mg/dL TIME : AM / PM
CORRECTED WITH:

NOTES

DATE: SUN MON TUES WED THUR FRI SAT

BREAKFAST	BLOOD SUGAR (BS): ____ TIME __:__ AM / PM Insulin Units: ____ mg/dL Total Carbs: ____ grams
MORNING SNACK	BLOOD SUGAR (BS): ____ TIME __:__ AM / PM Insulin Units: ____ mg/dL Total Carbs: ____ grams
LUNCH	BLOOD SUGAR (BS): ____ TIME __:__ AM / PM Insulin Units: ____ mg/dL Total Carbs: ____ grams
AFTERNOON SNACK	BLOOD SUGAR (BS): ____ TIME __:__ AM / PM Insulin Units: ____ mg/dL Total Carbs: ____ grams
DINNER	BLOOD SUGAR (BS): ____ TIME __:__ AM / PM Insulin Units: ____ mg/dL Total Carbs: ____ grams
EVENING SNACK	BLOOD SUGAR (BS): ____ TIME __:__ AM / PM Insulin Units: ____ mg/dL Total Carbs: ____ grams

BLOOD SUGAR HIGHS

TIME [:] AM / PM

BLOOD SUGAR (BS): [mg/dL]

CORRECTION DOSE: [units]

KETONES: NEGATIVE | TRACE | SMALL | MODERATE | LARGE

TIME [:] AM / PM

BLOOD SUGAR (BS): [mg/dL]

CORRECTION DOSE: [units]

KETONES: NEGATIVE | TRACE | SMALL | MODERATE | LARGE

TIME [:] AM / PM

BLOOD SUGAR (BS): [mg/dL]

CORRECTION DOSE: [units]

KETONES: NEGATIVE | TRACE | SMALL | MODERATE | LARGE

BLOOD SUGAR LOWS

BLOOD SUGAR (BS): [mg/dL] TIME [:] AM / PM

CORRECTED WITH: [ ]

BLOOD SUGAR (BS): [mg/dL] TIME [:] AM / PM

CORRECTED WITH: [ ]

NOTES

DATE: SUN MON TUES WED THUR FRI SAT

BREAKFAST

BLOOD SUGAR (BS): ______ TIME __ : __ AM / PM

Insulin Units: ______ mg/dL Total Carbs: ______ grams

MORNING SNACK

BLOOD SUGAR (BS): ______ TIME __ : __ AM / PM

Insulin Units: ______ mg/dL Total Carbs: ______ grams

LUNCH

BLOOD SUGAR (BS): ______ TIME __ : __ AM / PM

Insulin Units: ______ mg/dL Total Carbs: ______ grams

AFTERNOON SNACK

BLOOD SUGAR (BS): ______ TIME __ : __ AM / PM

Insulin Units: ______ mg/dL Total Carbs: ______ grams

DINNER

BLOOD SUGAR (BS): ______ TIME __ : __ AM / PM

Insulin Units: ______ mg/dL Total Carbs: ______ grams

EVENING SNACK

BLOOD SUGAR (BS): ______ TIME __ : __ AM / PM

Insulin Units: ______ mg/dL Total Carbs: ______ grams

BLOOD SUGAR HIGHS

TIME [:] AM / PM
BLOOD SUGAR (BS): [mg/dL]
CORRECTION DOSE: [units]

KETONES
NEGATIVE | TRACE | SMALL | MODERATE | LARGE

TIME [:] AM / PM
BLOOD SUGAR (BS): [mg/dL]
CORRECTION DOSE: [units]

KETONES
NEGATIVE | TRACE | SMALL | MODERATE | LARGE

TIME [:] AM / PM
BLOOD SUGAR (BS): [mg/dL]
CORRECTION DOSE: [units]

KETONES
NEGATIVE | TRACE | SMALL | MODERATE | LARGE

BLOOD SUGAR LOWS

BLOOD SUGAR (BS): [mg/dL] TIME [:] AM / PM
CORRECTED WITH:

BLOOD SUGAR (BS): [mg/dL] TIME [:] AM / PM
CORRECTED WITH:

NOTES

DATE: SUN MON TUES WED THUR FRI SAT

BREAKFAST

BLOOD SUGAR (BS): ______ TIME ___ : ___ AM / PM

Insulin Units: ______ mg/dL Total Carbs: ______ grams

MORNING SNACK

BLOOD SUGAR (BS): ______ TIME ___ : ___ AM / PM

Insulin Units: ______ mg/dL Total Carbs: ______ grams

LUNCH

BLOOD SUGAR (BS): ______ TIME ___ : ___ AM / PM

Insulin Units: ______ mg/dL Total Carbs: ______ grams

AFTERNOON SNACK

BLOOD SUGAR (BS): ______ TIME ___ : ___ AM / PM

Insulin Units: ______ mg/dL Total Carbs: ______ grams

DINNER

BLOOD SUGAR (BS): ______ TIME ___ : ___ AM / PM

Insulin Units: ______ mg/dL Total Carbs: ______ grams

EVENING SNACK

BLOOD SUGAR (BS): ______ TIME ___ : ___ AM / PM

Insulin Units: ______ mg/dL Total Carbs: ______ grams

BLOOD SUGAR HIGHS

TIME [:] AM / PM

BLOOD SUGAR (BS): [mg/dL]

CORRECTION DOSE: [units]

KETONES

NEGATIVE | TRACE | SMALL | MODERATE | LARGE

TIME [:] AM / PM

BLOOD SUGAR (BS): [mg/dL]

CORRECTION DOSE: [units]

KETONES

NEGATIVE | TRACE | SMALL | MODERATE | LARGE

TIME [:] AM / PM

BLOOD SUGAR (BS): [mg/dL]

CORRECTION DOSE: [units]

KETONES

NEGATIVE | TRACE | SMALL | MODERATE | LARGE

BLOOD SUGAR LOWS

BLOOD SUGAR (BS): [mg/dL] TIME [:] AM / PM

CORRECTED WITH: [ ]

BLOOD SUGAR (BS): [mg/dL] TIME [:] AM / PM

CORRECTED WITH: [ ]

NOTES

DATE: SUN MON TUES WED THUR FRI SAT

BREAKFAST	BLOOD SUGAR (BS): ______ TIME ___ : ___ AM / PM Insulin Units: ______ mg/dL Total Carbs: ______ grams
MORNING SNACK	BLOOD SUGAR (BS): ______ TIME ___ : ___ AM / PM Insulin Units: ______ mg/dL Total Carbs: ______ grams
LUNCH	BLOOD SUGAR (BS): ______ TIME ___ : ___ AM / PM Insulin Units: ______ mg/dL Total Carbs: ______ grams
AFTERNOON SNACK	BLOOD SUGAR (BS): ______ TIME ___ : ___ AM / PM Insulin Units: ______ mg/dL Total Carbs: ______ grams
DINNER	BLOOD SUGAR (BS): ______ TIME ___ : ___ AM / PM Insulin Units: ______ mg/dL Total Carbs: ______ grams
EVENING SNACK	BLOOD SUGAR (BS): ______ TIME ___ : ___ AM / PM Insulin Units: ______ mg/dL Total Carbs: ______ grams

BLOOD SUGAR HIGHS

TIME [:] AM / PM
BLOOD SUGAR (BS): [mg/dL]
CORRECTION DOSE: [units]

KETONES: NEGATIVE | TRACE | SMALL | MODERATE | LARGE

TIME [:] AM / PM
BLOOD SUGAR (BS): [mg/dL]
CORRECTION DOSE: [units]

KETONES: NEGATIVE | TRACE | SMALL | MODERATE | LARGE

TIME [:] AM / PM
BLOOD SUGAR (BS): [mg/dL]
CORRECTION DOSE: [units]

KETONES: NEGATIVE | TRACE | SMALL | MODERATE | LARGE

BLOOD SUGAR LOWS

BLOOD SUGAR (BS): [mg/dL] TIME [:] AM / PM
CORRECTED WITH: [ ]

BLOOD SUGAR (BS): [mg/dL] TIME [:] AM / PM
CORRECTED WITH: [ ]

NOTES

DATE: SUN MON TUES WED THUR FRI SAT

BREAKFAST	BLOOD SUGAR (BS): TIME : AM / PM Insulin Units: mg/dL Total Carbs: grams
MORNING SNACK	BLOOD SUGAR (BS): TIME : AM / PM Insulin Units: mg/dL Total Carbs: grams
LUNCH	BLOOD SUGAR (BS): TIME : AM / PM Insulin Units: mg/dL Total Carbs: grams
AFTERNOON SNACK	BLOOD SUGAR (BS): TIME : AM / PM Insulin Units: mg/dL Total Carbs: grams
DINNER	BLOOD SUGAR (BS): TIME : AM / PM Insulin Units: mg/dL Total Carbs: grams
EVENING SNACK	BLOOD SUGAR (BS): TIME : AM / PM Insulin Units: mg/dL Total Carbs: grams

BLOOD SUGAR HIGHS

TIME : AM / PM
BLOOD SUGAR (BS): mg/dL
CORRECTION DOSE: units

KETONES
NEGATIVE TRACE SMALL MODERATE LARGE

TIME : AM / PM
BLOOD SUGAR (BS): mg/dL
CORRECTION DOSE: units

KETONES
NEGATIVE TRACE SMALL MODERATE LARGE

TIME : AM / PM
BLOOD SUGAR (BS): mg/dL
CORRECTION DOSE: units

KETONES
NEGATIVE TRACE SMALL MODERATE LARGE

BLOOD SUGAR LOWS

BLOOD SUGAR (BS): mg/dL TIME : AM / PM
CORRECTED WITH:

BLOOD SUGAR (BS): mg/dL TIME : AM / PM
CORRECTED WITH:

NOTES

DATE: SUN MON TUES WED THUR FRI SAT

BREAKFAST	BLOOD SUGAR (BS): TIME : AM / PM Insulin Units: mg/dL Total Carbs: grams
MORNING SNACK	BLOOD SUGAR (BS): TIME : AM / PM Insulin Units: mg/dL Total Carbs: grams
LUNCH	BLOOD SUGAR (BS): TIME : AM / PM Insulin Units: mg/dL Total Carbs: grams
AFTERNOON SNACK	BLOOD SUGAR (BS): TIME : AM / PM Insulin Units: mg/dL Total Carbs: grams
DINNER	BLOOD SUGAR (BS): TIME : AM / PM Insulin Units: mg/dL Total Carbs: grams
EVENING SNACK	BLOOD SUGAR (BS): TIME : AM / PM Insulin Units: mg/dL Total Carbs: gams

BLOOD SUGAR HIGHS

TIME [:] AM / PM
BLOOD SUGAR (BS): [mg/dL]
CORRECTION DOSE: [units]

KETONES
NEGATIVE TRACE SMALL MODERATE LARGE

TIME [:] AM / PM
BLOOD SUGAR (BS): [mg/dL]
CORRECTION DOSE: [units]

KETONES
NEGATIVE TRACE SMALL MODERATE LARGE

TIME [:] AM / PM
BLOOD SUGAR (BS): [mg/dL]
CORRECTION DOSE: [units]

KETONES
NEGATIVE TRACE SMALL MODERATE LARGE

BLOOD SUGAR LOWS

BLOOD SUGAR (BS): [mg/dL] TIME [:] AM / PM
CORRECTED WITH:

BLOOD SUGAR (BS): [mg/dL] TIME [:] AM / PM
CORRECTED WITH:

NOTES

DATE: SUN MON TUES WED THUR FRI SAT

BREAKFAST	BLOOD SUGAR (BS): ____ TIME __:__ AM / PM Insulin Units: ____ mg/dL Total Carbs: ____ grams
MORNING SNACK	BLOOD SUGAR (BS): ____ TIME __:__ AM / PM Insulin Units: ____ mg/dL Total Carbs: ____ grams
LUNCH	BLOOD SUGAR (BS): ____ TIME __:__ AM / PM Insulin Units: ____ mg/dL Total Carbs: ____ grams
AFTERNOON SNACK	BLOOD SUGAR (BS): ____ TIME __:__ AM / PM Insulin Units: ____ mg/dL Total Carbs: ____ grams
DINNER	BLOOD SUGAR (BS): ____ TIME __:__ AM / PM Insulin Units: ____ mg/dL Total Carbs: ____ grams
EVENING SNACK	BLOOD SUGAR (BS): ____ TIME __:__ AM / PM Insulin Units: ____ mg/dL Total Carbs: ____ grams

BLOOD SUGAR HIGHS

TIME [:] AM / PM

BLOOD SUGAR (BS): [mg/dL]

CORRECTION DOSE: [units]

KETONES: NEGATIVE / TRACE / SMALL / MODERATE / LARGE

TIME [:] AM / PM

BLOOD SUGAR (BS): [mg/dL]

CORRECTION DOSE: [units]

KETONES: NEGATIVE / TRACE / SMALL / MODERATE / LARGE

TIME [:] AM / PM

BLOOD SUGAR (BS): [mg/dL]

CORRECTION DOSE: [units]

KETONES: NEGATIVE / TRACE / SMALL / MODERATE / LARGE

BLOOD SUGAR LOWS

BLOOD SUGAR (BS): [mg/dL] TIME [:] AM / PM

CORRECTED WITH:

BLOOD SUGAR (BS): [mg/dL] TIME [:] AM / PM

CORRECTED WITH:

NOTES

DATE: SUN MON TUES WED THUR FRI SAT

BREAKFAST	BLOOD SUGAR (BS): ____ TIME __ : __ AM / PM Insulin Units: ____ mg/dL Total Carbs: ____ grams
MORNING SNACK	BLOOD SUGAR (BS): ____ TIME __ : __ AM / PM Insulin Units: ____ mg/dL Total Carbs: ____ grams
LUNCH	BLOOD SUGAR (BS): ____ TIME __ : __ AM / PM Insulin Units: ____ mg/dL Total Carbs: ____ grams
AFTERNOON SNACK	BLOOD SUGAR (BS): ____ TIME __ : __ AM / PM Insulin Units: ____ mg/dL Total Carbs: ____ grams
DINNER	BLOOD SUGAR (BS): ____ TIME __ : __ AM / PM Insulin Units: ____ mg/dL Total Carbs: ____ grams
EVENING SNACK	BLOOD SUGAR (BS): ____ TIME __ : __ AM / PM Insulin Units: ____ mg/dL Total Carbs: ____ grams

BLOOD SUGAR HIGHS

TIME : AM / PM

BLOOD SUGAR (BS): mg/dL

CORRECTION DOSE: units

KETONES

NEGATIVE TRACE SMALL MODERATE LARGE

TIME : AM / PM

BLOOD SUGAR (BS): mg/dL

CORRECTION DOSE: units

KETONES

NEGATIVE TRACE SMALL MODERATE LARGE

TIME : AM / PM

BLOOD SUGAR (BS): mg/dL

CORRECTION DOSE: units

KETONES

NEGATIVE TRACE SMALL MODERATE LARGE

BLOOD SUGAR LOWS

BLOOD SUGAR (BS): mg/dL TIME : AM / PM

CORRECTED WITH:

BLOOD SUGAR (BS): mg/dL TIME : AM / PM

CORRECTED WITH:

NOTES

DATE: SUN MON TUES WED THUR FRI SAT

BREAKFAST	BLOOD SUGAR (BS): ____ TIME __:__ AM / PM Insulin Units: ____ mg/dL Total Carbs: ____ grams
MORNING SNACK	BLOOD SUGAR (BS): ____ TIME __:__ AM / PM Insulin Units: ____ mg/dL Total Carbs: ____ grams
LUNCH	BLOOD SUGAR (BS): ____ TIME __:__ AM / PM Insulin Units: ____ mg/dL Total Carbs: ____ grams
AFTERNOON SNACK	BLOOD SUGAR (BS): ____ TIME __:__ AM / PM Insulin Units: ____ mg/dL Total Carbs: ____ grams
DINNER	BLOOD SUGAR (BS): ____ TIME __:__ AM / PM Insulin Units: ____ mg/dL Total Carbs: ____ grams
EVENING SNACK	BLOOD SUGAR (BS): ____ TIME __:__ AM / PM Insulin Units: ____ mg/dL Total Carbs: ____ grams

BLOOD SUGAR HIGHS

TIME [:] AM / PM
BLOOD SUGAR (BS): [mg/dL]
CORRECTION DOSE: [units]

KETONES
NEGATIVE | TRACE | SMALL | MODERATE | LARGE

TIME [:] AM / PM
BLOOD SUGAR (BS): [mg/dL]
CORRECTION DOSE: [units]

KETONES
NEGATIVE | TRACE | SMALL | MODERATE | LARGE

TIME [:] AM / PM
BLOOD SUGAR (BS): [mg/dL]
CORRECTION DOSE: [units]

KETONES
NEGATIVE | TRACE | SMALL | MODERATE | LARGE

BLOOD SUGAR LOWS

BLOOD SUGAR (BS): [mg/dL] TIME [:] AM / PM
CORRECTED WITH: [ ]

BLOOD SUGAR (BS): [mg/dL] TIME [:] AM / PM
CORRECTED WITH: [ ]

NOTES

DATE: SUN MON TUES WED THUR FRI SAT

BREAKFAST

BLOOD SUGAR (BS): ______ TIME __:__ AM / PM

Insulin Units: ______ mg/dL Total Carbs: ______ grams

MORNING SNACK

BLOOD SUGAR (BS): ______ TIME __:__ AM / PM

Insulin Units: ______ mg/dL Total Carbs: ______ grams

LUNCH

BLOOD SUGAR (BS): ______ TIME __:__ AM / PM

Insulin Units: ______ mg/dL Total Carbs: ______ grams

AFTERNOON SNACK

BLOOD SUGAR (BS): ______ TIME __:__ AM / PM

Insulin Units: ______ mg/dL Total Carbs: ______ grams

DINNER

BLOOD SUGAR (BS): ______ TIME __:__ AM / PM

Insulin Units: ______ mg/dL Total Carbs: ______ grams

EVENING SNACK

BLOOD SUGAR (BS): ______ TIME __:__ AM / PM

Insulin Units: ______ mg/dL Total Carbs: ______ grams

BLOOD SUGAR HIGHS

TIME : AM / PM
BLOOD SUGAR (BS): mg/dL
CORRECTION DOSE: units

KETONES
NEGATIVE TRACE SMALL MODERATE LARGE

TIME : AM / PM
BLOOD SUGAR (BS): mg/dL
CORRECTION DOSE: units

KETONES
NEGATIVE TRACE SMALL MODERATE LARGE

TIME : AM / PM
BLOOD SUGAR (BS): mg/dL
CORRECTION DOSE: units

KETONES
NEGATIVE TRACE SMALL MODERATE LARGE

BLOOD SUGAR LOWS

BLOOD SUGAR (BS): mg/dL TIME : AM / PM
CORRECTED WITH:

BLOOD SUGAR (BS): mg/dL TIME : AM / PM
CORRECTED WITH:

NOTES

DATE: SUN MON TUES WED THUR FRI SAT

BREAKFAST

BLOOD SUGAR (BS): TIME : AM / PM

Insulin Units: mg/dL Total Carbs: grams

MORNING SNACK

BLOOD SUGAR (BS): TIME : AM / PM

Insulin Units: mg/dL Total Carbs: grams

LUNCH

BLOOD SUGAR (BS): TIME : AM / PM

Insulin Units: mg/dL Total Carbs: grams

AFTERNOON SNACK

BLOOD SUGAR (BS): TIME : AM / PM

Insulin Units: mg/dL Total Carbs: grams

DINNER

BLOOD SUGAR (BS): TIME : AM / PM

Insulin Units: mg/dL Total Carbs: grams

EVENING SNACK

BLOOD SUGAR (BS): TIME : AM / PM

Insulin Units: mg/dL Total Carbs: grams

BLOOD SUGAR HIGHS

TIME : AM / PM
BLOOD SUGAR (BS): mg/dL
CORRECTION DOSE: units

KETONES
NEGATIVE TRACE SMALL MODERATE LARGE

TIME : AM / PM
BLOOD SUGAR (BS): mg/dL
CORRECTION DOSE: units

KETONES
NEGATIVE TRACE SMALL MODERATE LARGE

TIME : AM / PM
BLOOD SUGAR (BS): mg/dL
CORRECTION DOSE: units

KETONES
NEGATIVE TRACE SMALL MODERATE LARGE

BLOOD SUGAR LOWS

BLOOD SUGAR (BS): mg/dL TIME : AM / PM
CORRECTED WITH:

BLOOD SUGAR (BS): mg/dL TIME : AM / PM
CORRECTED WITH:

NOTES

DATE: SUN MON TUES WED THUR FRI SAT

BREAKFAST

BLOOD SUGAR (BS): ______ TIME __ : __ AM / PM

Insulin Units: ______ mg/dL Total Carbs: ______ grams

MORNING SNACK

BLOOD SUGAR (BS): ______ TIME __ : __ AM / PM

Insulin Units: ______ mg/dL Total Carbs: ______ grams

LUNCH

BLOOD SUGAR (BS): ______ TIME __ : __ AM / PM

Insulin Units: ______ mg/dL Total Carbs: ______ grams

AFTERNOON SNACK

BLOOD SUGAR (BS): ______ TIME __ : __ AM / PM

Insulin Units: ______ mg/dL Total Carbs: ______ grams

DINNER

BLOOD SUGAR (BS): ______ TIME __ : __ AM / PM

Insulin Units: ______ mg/dL Total Carbs: ______ grams

EVENING SNACK

BLOOD SUGAR (BS): ______ TIME __ : __ AM / PM

Insulin Units: ______ mg/dL Total Carbs: ______ grams

BLOOD SUGAR HIGHS

TIME [:] AM / PM
BLOOD SUGAR (BS): [mg/dL]
CORRECTION DOSE: [units]

KETONES
NEGATIVE | TRACE | SMALL | MODERATE | LARGE

TIME [:] AM / PM
BLOOD SUGAR (BS): [mg/dL]
CORRECTION DOSE: [units]

KETONES
NEGATIVE | TRACE | SMALL | MODERATE | LARGE

TIME [:] AM / PM
BLOOD SUGAR (BS): [mg/dL]
CORRECTION DOSE: [units]

KETONES
NEGATIVE | TRACE | SMALL | MODERATE | LARGE

BLOOD SUGAR LOWS

BLOOD SUGAR (BS): [mg/dL] TIME [:] AM / PM
CORRECTED WITH:

BLOOD SUGAR (BS): [mg/dL] TIME [:] AM / PM
CORRECTED WITH:

NOTES

DATE: SUN MON TUES WED THUR FRI SAT

BREAKFAST

BLOOD SUGAR (BS): ______ TIME __ : __ AM / PM

Insulin Units: ______ mg/dL Total Carbs: ______ grams

MORNING SNACK

BLOOD SUGAR (BS): ______ TIME __ : __ AM / PM

Insulin Units: ______ mg/dL Total Carbs: ______ grams

LUNCH

BLOOD SUGAR (BS): ______ TIME __ : __ AM / PM

Insulin Units: ______ mg/dL Total Carbs: ______ grams

AFTERNOON SNACK

BLOOD SUGAR (BS): ______ TIME __ : __ AM / PM

Insulin Units: ______ mg/dL Total Carbs: ______ grams

DINNER

BLOOD SUGAR (BS): ______ TIME __ : __ AM / PM

Insulin Units: ______ mg/dL Total Carbs: ______ grams

EVENING SNACK

BLOOD SUGAR (BS): ______ TIME __ : __ AM / PM

Insulin Units: ______ mg/dL Total Carbs: ______ grams

BLOOD SUGAR HIGHS

TIME [:] AM / PM

BLOOD SUGAR (BS): [mg/dL]

CORRECTION DOSE: units

KETONES: NEGATIVE · TRACE · SMALL · MODERATE · LARGE

TIME [:] AM / PM

BLOOD SUGAR (BS): [mg/dL]

CORRECTION DOSE: units

KETONES: NEGATIVE · TRACE · SMALL · MODERATE · LARGE

TIME [:] AM / PM

BLOOD SUGAR (BS): [mg/dL]

CORRECTION DOSE: units

KETONES: NEGATIVE · TRACE · SMALL · MODERATE · LARGE

BLOOD SUGAR LOWS

BLOOD SUGAR (BS): [mg/dL] TIME [:] AM / PM

CORRECTED WITH:

BLOOD SUGAR (BS): [mg/dL] TIME [:] AM / PM

CORRECTED WITH:

NOTES

DATE: SUN MON TUES WED THUR FRI SAT

BREAKFAST

BLOOD SUGAR (BS): ______ TIME __:__ AM / PM

Insulin Units: ______ mg/dL Total Carbs: ______ grams

MORNING SNACK

BLOOD SUGAR (BS): ______ TIME __:__ AM / PM

Insulin Units: ______ mg/dL Total Carbs: ______ grams

LUNCH

BLOOD SUGAR (BS): ______ TIME __:__ AM / PM

Insulin Units: ______ mg/dL Total Carbs: ______ grams

AFTERNOON SNACK

BLOOD SUGAR (BS): ______ TIME __:__ AM / PM

Insulin Units: ______ mg/dL Total Carbs: ______ grams

DINNER

BLOOD SUGAR (BS): ______ TIME __:__ AM / PM

Insulin Units: ______ mg/dL Total Carbs: ______ grams

EVENING SNACK

BLOOD SUGAR (BS): ______ TIME __:__ AM / PM

Insulin Units: ______ mg/dL Total Carbs: ______ grams

BLOOD SUGAR HIGHS

TIME [:] AM / PM
BLOOD SUGAR (BS): [mg/dL]
CORRECTION DOSE: [units]

KETONES
NEGATIVE | TRACE | SMALL | MODERATE | LARGE

TIME [:] AM / PM
BLOOD SUGAR (BS): [mg/dL]
CORRECTION DOSE: [units]

KETONES
NEGATIVE | TRACE | SMALL | MODERATE | LARGE

TIME [:] AM / PM
BLOOD SUGAR (BS): [mg/dL]
CORRECTION DOSE: [units]

KETONES
NEGATIVE | TRACE | SMALL | MODERATE | LARGE

BLOOD SUGAR LOWS

BLOOD SUGAR (BS): [mg/dL] TIME [:] AM / PM
CORRECTED WITH: [ ]

BLOOD SUGAR (BS): [mg/dL] TIME [:] AM / PM
CORRECTED WITH: [ ]

NOTES

DATE: SUN MON TUES WED THUR FRI SAT

BREAKFAST

BLOOD SUGAR (BS): TIME : AM / PM

Insulin Units: mg/dL Total Carbs: grams

MORNING SNACK

BLOOD SUGAR (BS): TIME : AM / PM

Insulin Units: mg/dL Total Carbs: grams

LUNCH

BLOOD SUGAR (BS): TIME : AM / PM

Insulin Units: mg/dL Total Carbs: grams

AFTERNOON SNACK

BLOOD SUGAR (BS): TIME : AM / PM

Insulin Units: mg/dL Total Carbs: grams

DINNER

BLOOD SUGAR (BS): TIME : AM / PM

Insulin Units: mg/dL Total Carbs: grams

EVENING SNACK

BLOOD SUGAR (BS): TIME : AM / PM

Insulin Units: mg/dL Total Carbs: grams

BLOOD SUGAR HIGHS

TIME : AM / PM

BLOOD SUGAR (BS): mg/dL

CORRECTION DOSE: units

KETONES

NEGATIVE TRACE SMALL MODERATE LARGE

TIME : AM / PM

BLOOD SUGAR (BS): mg/dL

CORRECTION DOSE: units

KETONES

NEGATIVE TRACE SMALL MODERATE LARGE

TIME : AM / PM

BLOOD SUGAR (BS): mg/dL

CORRECTION DOSE: units

KETONES

NEGATIVE TRACE SMALL MODERATE LARGE

BLOOD SUGAR LOWS

BLOOD SUGAR (BS): mg/dL TIME : AM / PM

CORRECTED WITH:

BLOOD SUGAR (BS): mg/dL TIME : AM / PM

CORRECTED WITH:

NOTES

DATE: SUN MON TUES WED THUR FRI SAT

BREAKFAST

BLOOD SUGAR (BS): TIME : AM / PM

Insulin Units: mg/dL Total Carbs: grams

MORNING SNACK

BLOOD SUGAR (BS): TIME : AM / PM

Insulin Units: mg/dL Total Carbs: grams

LUNCH

BLOOD SUGAR (BS): TIME : AM / PM

Insulin Units: mg/dL Total Carbs: grams

AFTERNOON SNACK

BLOOD SUGAR (BS): TIME : AM / PM

Insulin Units: mg/dL Total Carbs: grams

DINNER

BLOOD SUGAR (BS): TIME : AM / PM

Insulin Units: mg/dL Total Carbs: grams

EVENING SNACK

BLOOD SUGAR (BS): TIME : AM / PM

Insulin Units: mg/dL Total Carbs: grams

BLOOD SUGAR HIGHS

TIME [:] AM / PM
BLOOD SUGAR (BS): [mg/dL]
CORRECTION DOSE: [units]

KETONES: NEGATIVE / TRACE / SMALL / MODERATE / LARGE

TIME [:] AM / PM
BLOOD SUGAR (BS): [mg/dL]
CORRECTION DOSE: [units]

KETONES: NEGATIVE / TRACE / SMALL / MODERATE / LARGE

TIME [:] AM / PM
BLOOD SUGAR (BS): [mg/dL]
CORRECTION DOSE: [units]

KETONES: NEGATIVE / TRACE / SMALL / MODERATE / LARGE

BLOOD SUGAR LOWS

BLOOD SUGAR (BS): [mg/dL] TIME [:] AM / PM
CORRECTED WITH:

BLOOD SUGAR (BS): [mg/dL] TIME [:] AM / PM
CORRECTED WITH:

NOTES

DATE: SUN MON TUES WED THUR FRI SAT

BREAKFAST

BLOOD SUGAR (BS): ______ TIME ___ : ___ AM / PM

Insulin Units: ______ mg/dL Total Carbs: ______ grams

MORNING SNACK

BLOOD SUGAR (BS): ______ TIME ___ : ___ AM / PM

Insulin Units: ______ mg/dL Total Carbs: ______ grams

LUNCH

BLOOD SUGAR (BS): ______ TIME ___ : ___ AM / PM

Insulin Units: ______ mg/dL Total Carbs: ______ grams

AFTERNOON SNACK

BLOOD SUGAR (BS): ______ TIME ___ : ___ AM / PM

Insulin Units: ______ mg/dL Total Carbs: ______ grams

DINNER

BLOOD SUGAR (BS): ______ TIME ___ : ___ AM / PM

Insulin Units: ______ mg/dL Total Carbs: ______ grams

EVENING SNACK

BLOOD SUGAR (BS): ______ TIME ___ : ___ AM / PM

Insulin Units: ______ mg/dL Total Carbs: ______ grams

BLOOD SUGAR HIGHS

TIME : AM / PM
BLOOD SUGAR (BS): mg/dL
CORRECTION DOSE: units

KETONES
NEGATIVE TRACE SMALL MODERATE LARGE

TIME : AM / PM
BLOOD SUGAR (BS): mg/dL
CORRECTION DOSE: units

KETONES
NEGATIVE TRACE SMALL MODERATE LARGE

TIME : AM / PM
BLOOD SUGAR (BS): mg/dL
CORRECTION DOSE: units

KETONES
NEGATIVE TRACE SMALL MODERATE LARGE

BLOOD SUGAR LOWS

BLOOD SUGAR (BS): mg/dL TIME : AM / PM
CORRECTED WITH:

BLOOD SUGAR (BS): mg/dL TIME : AM / PM
CORRECTED WITH:

NOTES

DATE: SUN MON TUES WED THUR FRI SAT

BREAKFAST

BLOOD SUGAR (BS): TIME : AM / PM

Insulin Units: mg/dL Total Carbs: grams

MORNING SNACK

BLOOD SUGAR (BS): TIME : AM / PM

Insulin Units: mg/dL Total Carbs: grams

LUNCH

BLOOD SUGAR (BS): TIME : AM / PM

Insulin Units: mg/dL Total Carbs: grams

AFTERNOON SNACK

BLOOD SUGAR (BS): TIME : AM / PM

Insulin Units: mg/dL Total Carbs: grams

DINNER

BLOOD SUGAR (BS): TIME : AM / PM

Insulin Units: mg/dL Total Carbs: grams

EVENING SNACK

BLOOD SUGAR (BS): TIME : AM / PM

Insulin Units: mg/dL Total Carbs: grams

BLOOD SUGAR HIGHS

TIME : AM / PM

BLOOD SUGAR (BS): mg/dL

CORRECTION DOSE: units

KETONES

NEGATIVE TRACE SMALL MODERATE LARGE

TIME : AM / PM

BLOOD SUGAR (BS): mg/dL

CORRECTION DOSE: units

KETONES

NEGATIVE TRACE SMALL MODERATE LARGE

TIME : AM / PM

BLOOD SUGAR (BS): mg/dL

CORRECTION DOSE: units

KETONES

NEGATIVE TRACE SMALL MODERATE LARGE

BLOOD SUGAR LOWS

BLOOD SUGAR (BS): mg/dL TIME : AM / PM

CORRECTED WITH:

BLOOD SUGAR (BS): mg/dL TIME : AM / PM

CORRECTED WITH:

NOTES

DATE: SUN MON TUES WED THUR FRI SAT

BREAKFAST

BLOOD SUGAR (BS): ______ TIME ___ : ___ AM / PM

Insulin Units: ______ mg/dL Total Carbs: ______ grams

MORNING SNACK

BLOOD SUGAR (BS): ______ TIME ___ : ___ AM / PM

Insulin Units: ______ mg/dL Total Carbs: ______ grams

LUNCH

BLOOD SUGAR (BS): ______ TIME ___ : ___ AM / PM

Insulin Units: ______ mg/dL Total Carbs: ______ grams

AFTERNOON SNACK

BLOOD SUGAR (BS): ______ TIME ___ : ___ AM / PM

Insulin Units: ______ mg/dL Total Carbs: ______ grams

DINNER

BLOOD SUGAR (BS): ______ TIME ___ : ___ AM / PM

Insulin Units: ______ mg/dL Total Carbs: ______ grams

EVENING SNACK

BLOOD SUGAR (BS): ______ TIME ___ : ___ AM / PM

Insulin Units: ______ mg/dL Total Carbs: ______ grams

BLOOD SUGAR HIGHS

TIME : AM / PM
BLOOD SUGAR (BS): mg/dL
CORRECTION DOSE: units

KETONES
NEGATIVE TRACE SMALL MODERATE LARGE

TIME : AM / PM
BLOOD SUGAR (BS): mg/dL
CORRECTION DOSE: units

KETONES
NEGATIVE TRACE SMALL MODERATE LARGE

TIME : AM / PM
BLOOD SUGAR (BS): mg/dL
CORRECTION DOSE: units

KETONES
NEGATIVE TRACE SMALL MODERATE LARGE

BLOOD SUGAR LOWS

BLOOD SUGAR (BS): mg/dL TIME : AM / PM
CORRECTED WITH:

BLOOD SUGAR (BS): mg/dL TIME : AM / PM
CORRECTED WITH:

NOTES

DATE: SUN MON TUES WED THUR FRI SAT

BREAKFAST

BLOOD SUGAR (BS): TIME : AM / PM

Insulin Units: mg/dL Total Carbs: grams

MORNING SNACK

BLOOD SUGAR (BS): TIME : AM / PM

Insulin Units: mg/dL Total Carbs: grams

LUNCH

BLOOD SUGAR (BS): TIME : AM / PM

Insulin Units: mg/dL Total Carbs: grams

AFTERNOON SNACK

BLOOD SUGAR (BS): TIME : AM / PM

Insulin Units: mg/dL Total Carbs: grams

DINNER

BLOOD SUGAR (BS): TIME : AM / PM

Insulin Units: mg/dL Total Carbs: grams

EVENING SNACK

BLOOD SUGAR (BS): TIME : AM / PM

Insulin Units: mg/dL Total Carbs: grams

BLOOD SUGAR HIGHS

TIME : AM / PM

BLOOD SUGAR (BS): mg/dL

CORRECTION DOSE: units

KETONES

NEGATIVE TRACE SMALL MODERATE LARGE

TIME : AM / PM

BLOOD SUGAR (BS): mg/dL

CORRECTION DOSE: units

KETONES

NEGATIVE TRACE SMALL MODERATE LARGE

TIME : AM / PM

BLOOD SUGAR (BS): mg/dL

CORRECTION DOSE: units

KETONES

NEGATIVE TRACE SMALL MODERATE LARGE

BLOOD SUGAR LOWS

BLOOD SUGAR (BS): mg/dL TIME : AM / PM

CORRECTED WITH:

BLOOD SUGAR (BS): mg/dL TIME : AM / PM

CORRECTED WITH:

NOTES

DATE: SUN MON TUES WED THUR FRI SAT

BREAKFAST

BLOOD SUGAR (BS): TIME : AM / PM

Insulin Units: mg/dL Total Carbs: grams

MORNING SNACK

BLOOD SUGAR (BS): TIME : AM / PM

Insulin Units: mg/dL Total Carbs: grams

LUNCH

BLOOD SUGAR (BS): TIME : AM / PM

Insulin Units: mg/dL Total Carbs: grams

AFTERNOON SNACK

BLOOD SUGAR (BS): TIME : AM / PM

Insulin Units: mg/dL Total Carbs: grams

DINNER

BLOOD SUGAR (BS): TIME : AM / PM

Insulin Units: mg/dL Total Carbs: grams

EVENING SNACK

BLOOD SUGAR (BS): TIME : AM / PM

Insulin Units: mg/dL Total Carbs: grams

BLOOD SUGAR HIGHS

TIME : AM / PM
BLOOD SUGAR (BS): mg/dL
CORRECTION DOSE: units

KETONES
NEGATIVE TRACE SMALL MODERATE LARGE

TIME : AM / PM
BLOOD SUGAR (BS): mg/dL
CORRECTION DOSE: units

KETONES
NEGATIVE TRACE SMALL MODERATE LARGE

TIME : AM / PM
BLOOD SUGAR (BS): mg/dL
CORRECTION DOSE: units

KETONES
NEGATIVE TRACE SMALL MODERATE LARGE

BLOOD SUGAR LOWS

BLOOD SUGAR (BS): mg/dL TIME : AM / PM
CORRECTED WITH:

BLOOD SUGAR (BS): mg/dL TIME : AM / PM
CORRECTED WITH:

NOTES

DATE: SUN MON TUES WED THUR FRI SAT

BREAKFAST	BLOOD SUGAR (BS): TIME : AM / PM Insulin Units: mg/dL Total Carbs: grams
MORNING SNACK	BLOOD SUGAR (BS): TIME : AM / PM Insulin Units: mg/dL Total Carbs: grams
LUNCH	BLOOD SUGAR (BS): TIME : AM / PM Insulin Units: mg/dL Total Carbs: grams
AFTERNOON SNACK	BLOOD SUGAR (BS): TIME : AM / PM Insulin Units: mg/dL Total Carbs: grams
DINNER	BLOOD SUGAR (BS): TIME : AM / PM Insulin Units: mg/dL Total Carbs: grams
EVENING SNACK	BLOOD SUGAR (BS): TIME : AM / PM Insulin Units: mg/dL Total Carbs: grams

BLOOD SUGAR HIGHS

TIME : AM / PM

BLOOD SUGAR (BS): mg/dL

CORRECTION DOSE: units

KETONES

NEGATIVE TRACE SMALL MODERATE LARGE

TIME : AM / PM

BLOOD SUGAR (BS): mg/dL

CORRECTION DOSE: units

KETONES

NEGATIVE TRACE SMALL MODERATE LARGE

TIME : AM / PM

BLOOD SUGAR (BS): mg/dL

CORRECTION DOSE: units

KETONES

NEGATIVE TRACE SMALL MODERATE LARGE

BLOOD SUGAR LOWS

BLOOD SUGAR (BS): mg/dL TIME : AM / PM

CORRECTED WITH:

BLOOD SUGAR (BS): mg/dL TIME : AM / PM

CORRECTED WITH:

NOTES

DATE: SUN MON TUES WED THUR FRI SAT

BREAKFAST

BLOOD SUGAR (BS): ______ TIME __ : __ AM / PM

Insulin Units: ______ mg/dL Total Carbs: ______ grams

MORNING SNACK

BLOOD SUGAR (BS): ______ TIME __ : __ AM / PM

Insulin Units: ______ mg/dL Total Carbs: ______ grams

LUNCH

BLOOD SUGAR (BS): ______ TIME __ : __ AM / PM

Insulin Units: ______ mg/dL Total Carbs: ______ grams

AFTERNOON SNACK

BLOOD SUGAR (BS): ______ TIME __ : __ AM / PM

Insulin Units: ______ mg/dL Total Carbs: ______ grams

DINNER

BLOOD SUGAR (BS): ______ TIME __ : __ AM / PM

Insulin Units: ______ mg/dL Total Carbs: ______ grams

EVENING SNACK

BLOOD SUGAR (BS): ______ TIME __ : __ AM / PM

Insulin Units: ______ mg/dL Total Carbs: ______ grams

BLOOD SUGAR HIGHS

TIME : AM / PM

BLOOD SUGAR (BS): mg/dL

CORRECTION DOSE: units

KETONES

NEGATIVE TRACE SMALL MODERATE LARGE

TIME : AM / PM

BLOOD SUGAR (BS): mg/dL

CORRECTION DOSE: units

KETONES

NEGATIVE TRACE SMALL MODERATE LARGE

TIME : AM / PM

BLOOD SUGAR (BS): mg/dL

CORRECTION DOSE: units

KETONES

NEGATIVE TRACE SMALL MODERATE LARGE

BLOOD SUGAR LOWS

BLOOD SUGAR (BS): mg/dL TIME : AM / PM

CORRECTED WITH:

BLOOD SUGAR (BS): mg/dL TIME : AM / PM

CORRECTED WITH:

NOTES

DATE: SUN MON TUES WED THUR FRI SAT

BREAKFAST

BLOOD SUGAR (BS): TIME : AM / PM

Insulin Units: mg/dL Total Carbs: grams

MORNING SNACK

BLOOD SUGAR (BS): TIME : AM / PM

Insulin Units: mg/dL Total Carbs: grams

LUNCH

BLOOD SUGAR (BS): TIME : AM / PM

Insulin Units: mg/dL Total Carbs: grams

AFTERNOON SNACK

BLOOD SUGAR (BS): TIME : AM / PM

Insulin Units: mg/dL Total Carbs: grams

DINNER

BLOOD SUGAR (BS): TIME : AM / PM

Insulin Units: mg/dL Total Carbs: grams

EVENING SNACK

BLOOD SUGAR (BS): TIME : AM / PM

Insulin Units: mg/dL Total Carbs: grams

BLOOD SUGAR HIGHS

TIME : AM / PM

BLOOD SUGAR (BS): mg/dL

CORRECTION DOSE: units

KETONES

NEGATIVE TRACE SMALL MODERATE LARGE

TIME : AM / PM

BLOOD SUGAR (BS): mg/dL

CORRECTION DOSE: units

KETONES

NEGATIVE TRACE SMALL MODERATE LARGE

TIME : AM / PM

BLOOD SUGAR (BS): mg/dL

CORRECTION DOSE: units

KETONES

NEGATIVE TRACE SMALL MODERATE LARGE

BLOOD SUGAR LOWS

BLOOD SUGAR (BS): mg/dL TIME : AM / PM

CORRECTED WITH:

BLOOD SUGAR (BS): mg/dL TIME : AM / PM

CORRECTED WITH:

NOTES

DATE: SUN MON TUES WED THUR FRI SAT

BREAKFAST	BLOOD SUGAR (BS): ____ TIME __ : __ AM / PM Insulin Units: ____ mg/dL Total Carbs: ____ grams
MORNING SNACK	BLOOD SUGAR (BS): ____ TIME __ : __ AM / PM Insulin Units: ____ mg/dL Total Carbs: ____ grams
LUNCH	BLOOD SUGAR (BS): ____ TIME __ : __ AM / PM Insulin Units: ____ mg/dL Total Carbs: ____ grams
AFTERNOON SNACK	BLOOD SUGAR (BS): ____ TIME __ : __ AM / PM Insulin Units: ____ mg/dL Total Carbs: ____ grams
DINNER	BLOOD SUGAR (BS): ____ TIME __ : __ AM / PM Insulin Units: ____ mg/dL Total Carbs: ____ grams
EVENING SNACK	BLOOD SUGAR (BS): ____ TIME __ : __ AM / PM Insulin Units: ____ mg/dL Total Carbs: ____ grams

BLOOD SUGAR HIGHS

TIME : AM / PM
BLOOD SUGAR (BS): mg/dL
CORRECTION DOSE: units
KETONES: NEGATIVE · TRACE · SMALL · MODERATE · LARGE

TIME : AM / PM
BLOOD SUGAR (BS): mg/dL
CORRECTION DOSE: units
KETONES: NEGATIVE · TRACE · SMALL · MODERATE · LARGE

TIME : AM / PM
BLOOD SUGAR (BS): mg/dL
CORRECTION DOSE: units
KETONES: NEGATIVE · TRACE · SMALL · MODERATE · LARGE

BLOOD SUGAR LOWS

BLOOD SUGAR (BS): mg/dL TIME : AM / PM
CORRECTED WITH:

BLOOD SUGAR (BS): mg/dL TIME : AM / PM
CORRECTED WITH:

NOTES

DATE: SUN MON TUES WED THUR FRI SAT

BREAKFAST	BLOOD SUGAR (BS): TIME : AM / PM Insulin Units: mg/dL Total Carbs: grams
MORNING SNACK	BLOOD SUGAR (BS): TIME : AM / PM Insulin Units: mg/dL Total Carbs: grams
LUNCH	BLOOD SUGAR (BS): TIME : AM / PM Insulin Units: mg/dL Total Carbs: grams
AFTERNOON SNACK	BLOOD SUGAR (BS): TIME : AM / PM Insulin Units: mg/dL Total Carbs: grams
DINNER	BLOOD SUGAR (BS): TIME : AM / PM Insulin Units: mg/dL Total Carbs: grams
EVENING SNACK	BLOOD SUGAR (BS): TIME : AM / PM Insulin Units: mg/dL Total Carbs: grams

BLOOD SUGAR HIGHS

TIME : AM / PM
BLOOD SUGAR (BS): mg/dL
CORRECTION DOSE: units

KETONES
NEGATIVE TRACE SMALL MODERATE LARGE

TIME : AM / PM
BLOOD SUGAR (BS): mg/dL
CORRECTION DOSE: units

KETONES
NEGATIVE TRACE SMALL MODERATE LARGE

TIME : AM / PM
BLOOD SUGAR (BS): mg/dL
CORRECTION DOSE: units

KETONES
NEGATIVE TRACE SMALL MODERATE LARGE

BLOOD SUGAR LOWS

BLOOD SUGAR (BS): mg/dL TIME : AM / PM
CORRECTED WITH:

BLOOD SUGAR (BS): mg/dL TIME : AM / PM
CORRECTED WITH:

NOTES

DATE: SUN MON TUES WED THUR FRI SAT

BREAKFAST

BLOOD SUGAR (BS): ______ TIME ___ : ___ AM / PM

Insulin Units: ______ mg/dL Total Carbs: ______ grams

MORNING SNACK

BLOOD SUGAR (BS): ______ TIME ___ : ___ AM / PM

Insulin Units: ______ mg/dL Total Carbs: ______ grams

LUNCH

BLOOD SUGAR (BS): ______ TIME ___ : ___ AM / PM

Insulin Units: ______ mg/dL Total Carbs: ______ grams

AFTERNOON SNACK

BLOOD SUGAR (BS): ______ TIME ___ : ___ AM / PM

Insulin Units: ______ mg/dL Total Carbs: ______ grams

DINNER

BLOOD SUGAR (BS): ______ TIME ___ : ___ AM / PM

Insulin Units: ______ mg/dL Total Carbs: ______ grams

EVENING SNACK

BLOOD SUGAR (BS): ______ TIME ___ : ___ AM / PM

Insulin Units: ______ mg/dL Total Carbs: ______ grams

BLOOD SUGAR HIGHS

TIME : AM / PM
BLOOD SUGAR (BS): mg/dL
CORRECTION DOSE: units

KETONES
NEGATIVE TRACE SMALL MODERATE LARGE

TIME : AM / PM
BLOOD SUGAR (BS): mg/dL
CORRECTION DOSE: units

KETONES
NEGATIVE TRACE SMALL MODERATE LARGE

TIME : AM / PM
BLOOD SUGAR (BS): mg/dL
CORRECTION DOSE: units

KETONES
NEGATIVE TRACE SMALL MODERATE LARGE

BLOOD SUGAR LOWS

BLOOD SUGAR (BS): mg/dL TIME : AM / PM
CORRECTED WITH:

BLOOD SUGAR (BS): mg/dL TIME : AM / PM
CORRECTED WITH:

NOTES

DATE: SUN MON TUES WED THUR FRI SAT

BREAKFAST

BLOOD SUGAR (BS): ______ TIME ___:___ AM / PM

Insulin Units: ______ mg/dL Total Carbs: ______ grams

MORNING SNACK

BLOOD SUGAR (BS): ______ TIME ___:___ AM / PM

Insulin Units: ______ mg/dL Total Carbs: ______ grams

LUNCH

BLOOD SUGAR (BS): ______ TIME ___:___ AM / PM

Insulin Units: ______ mg/dL Total Carbs: ______ grams

AFTERNOON SNACK

BLOOD SUGAR (BS): ______ TIME ___:___ AM / PM

Insulin Units: ______ mg/dL Total Carbs: ______ grams

DINNER

BLOOD SUGAR (BS): ______ TIME ___:___ AM / PM

Insulin Units: ______ mg/dL Total Carbs: ______ grams

EVENING SNACK

BLOOD SUGAR (BS): ______ TIME ___:___ AM / PM

Insulin Units: ______ mg/dL Total Carbs: ______ grams

BLOOD SUGAR HIGHS

TIME : AM / PM
BLOOD SUGAR (BS): mg/dL
CORRECTION DOSE: units

KETONES
NEGATIVE TRACE SMALL MODERATE LARGE

TIME : AM / PM
BLOOD SUGAR (BS): mg/dL
CORRECTION DOSE: units

KETONES
NEGATIVE TRACE SMALL MODERATE LARGE

TIME : AM / PM
BLOOD SUGAR (BS): mg/dL
CORRECTION DOSE: units

KETONES
NEGATIVE TRACE SMALL MODERATE LARGE

BLOOD SUGAR LOWS

BLOOD SUGAR (BS): mg/dL TIME : AM / PM
CORRECTED WITH:

BLOOD SUGAR (BS): mg/dL TIME : AM / PM
CORRECTED WITH:

NOTES

DATE: SUN MON TUES WED THUR FRI SAT

BREAKFAST	BLOOD SUGAR (BS): TIME : AM / PM Insulin Units: mg/dL Total Carbs: grams
MORNING SNACK	BLOOD SUGAR (BS): TIME : AM / PM Insulin Units: mg/dL Total Carbs: grams
LUNCH	BLOOD SUGAR (BS): TIME : AM / PM Insulin Units: mg/dL Total Carbs: grams
AFTERNOON SNACK	BLOOD SUGAR (BS): TIME : AM / PM Insulin Units: mg/dL Total Carbs: grams
DINNER	BLOOD SUGAR (BS): TIME : AM / PM Insulin Units: mg/dL Total Carbs: grams
EVENING SNACK	BLOOD SUGAR (BS): TIME : AM / PM Insulin Units: mg/dL Total Carbs: grams

BLOOD SUGAR HIGHS

TIME [:] AM / PM
BLOOD SUGAR (BS): [mg/dL]
CORRECTION DOSE: [units]

KETONES
NEGATIVE TRACE SMALL MODERATE LARGE

TIME [:] AM / PM
BLOOD SUGAR (BS): [mg/dL]
CORRECTION DOSE: [units]

KETONES
NEGATIVE TRACE SMALL MODERATE LARGE

TIME [:] AM / PM
BLOOD SUGAR (BS): [mg/dL]
CORRECTION DOSE: [units]

KETONES
NEGATIVE TRACE SMALL MODERATE LARGE

BLOOD SUGAR LOWS

BLOOD SUGAR (BS): [mg/dL] TIME [:] AM / PM
CORRECTED WITH:

BLOOD SUGAR (BS): [mg/dL] TIME [:] AM / PM
CORRECTED WITH:

NOTES

DATE: SUN MON TUES WED THUR FRI SAT

BREAKFAST	BLOOD SUGAR (BS): TIME : AM / PM Insulin Units: mg/dL Total Carbs: grams
MORNING SNACK	BLOOD SUGAR (BS): TIME : AM / PM Insulin Units: mg/dL Total Carbs: grams
LUNCH	BLOOD SUGAR (BS): TIME : AM / PM Insulin Units: mg/dL Total Carbs: grams
AFTERNOON SNACK	BLOOD SUGAR (BS): TIME : AM / PM Insulin Units: mg/dL Total Carbs: grams
DINNER	BLOOD SUGAR (BS): TIME : AM / PM Insulin Units: mg/dL Total Carbs: grams
EVENING SNACK	BLOOD SUGAR (BS): TIME : AM / PM Insulin Units: mg/dL Total Carbs: grams

BLOOD SUGAR HIGHS

TIME : AM / PM
BLOOD SUGAR (BS): mg/dL
CORRECTION DOSE: units

KETONES
NEGATIVE TRACE SMALL MODERATE LARGE

TIME : AM / PM
BLOOD SUGAR (BS): mg/dL
CORRECTION DOSE: units

KETONES
NEGATIVE TRACE SMALL MODERATE LARGE

TIME : AM / PM
BLOOD SUGAR (BS): mg/dL
CORRECTION DOSE: units

KETONES
NEGATIVE TRACE SMALL MODERATE LARGE

BLOOD SUGAR LOWS

BLOOD SUGAR (BS): mg/dL TIME : AM / PM
CORRECTED WITH:

BLOOD SUGAR (BS): mg/dL TIME : AM / PM
CORRECTED WITH:

NOTES

DATE: SUN MON TUES WED THUR FRI SAT

BREAKFAST

BLOOD SUGAR (BS): ______ TIME ___:___ AM / PM

Insulin Units: ______ mg/dL Total Carbs: ______ grams

MORNING SNACK

BLOOD SUGAR (BS): ______ TIME ___:___ AM / PM

Insulin Units: ______ mg/dL Total Carbs: ______ grams

LUNCH

BLOOD SUGAR (BS): ______ TIME ___:___ AM / PM

Insulin Units: ______ mg/dL Total Carbs: ______ grams

AFTERNOON SNACK

BLOOD SUGAR (BS): ______ TIME ___:___ AM / PM

Insulin Units: ______ mg/dL Total Carbs: ______ grams

DINNER

BLOOD SUGAR (BS): ______ TIME ___:___ AM / PM

Insulin Units: ______ mg/dL Total Carbs: ______ grams

EVENING SNACK

BLOOD SUGAR (BS): ______ TIME ___:___ AM / PM

Insulin Units: ______ mg/dL Total Carbs: ______ grams

BLOOD SUGAR HIGHS

TIME : AM / PM
BLOOD SUGAR (BS): mg/dL
CORRECTION DOSE: units

KETONES
NEGATIVE TRACE SMALL MODERATE LARGE

TIME : AM / PM
BLOOD SUGAR (BS): mg/dL
CORRECTION DOSE: units

KETONES
NEGATIVE TRACE SMALL MODERATE LARGE

TIME : AM / PM
BLOOD SUGAR (BS): mg/dL
CORRECTION DOSE: units

KETONES
NEGATIVE TRACE SMALL MODERATE LARGE

BLOOD SUGAR LOWS

BLOOD SUGAR (BS): mg/dL TIME : AM / PM
CORRECTED WITH:

BLOOD SUGAR (BS): mg/dL TIME : AM / PM
CORRECTED WITH:

NOTES

NOTES

NOTES

NOTES

NOTES

NOTES

NOTES

NOTES

NOTES

Made in the USA
Monee, IL
03 November 2026

67386125R00046